The Obesity Remedy

Uncovering the Mysteries of Weight Loss

By

Kevin Alex Malkovic

U.S. and worldwide. This tendency will likely continue to drive the global obesity pandemic for decades, affecting population health, posing infrastructure issues as governments strive to fulfil the increased healthcare needs, and dramatically raising healthcare costs worldwide.

Beyond personal weight management, social and economic innovations will be essential that concentrate on methods to avoid further rises in overweight and obesity rates.

Unwanted weight gain resulting in overweight and obesity has become a primary cause of the worldwide increase in non-communicable illnesses and is now considered a non-communicable disease. Because of the psychological and social stigmata that precede being overweight and obese, persons suffering from these disorders are also subject to discrimination in their personal and professional life, poor self-esteem, and despair. These physiological and psychological repercussions of obesity contribute to a substantial part of current healthcare expenses and cause extra economic costs via loss of output per worker, increased disability, and early loss of life.

The recognition that being overweight or obese is a chronic disease and not simply due to poor self-control, or a total absence of willpower comes from the past 70 years of research that has been rapidly gaining insight into the physiology that controls body weight (homeostatic mechanisms involved in sensing and adapting to changes in the body's internal metabolism, environmental availability of food, and activity levels to maintain body weight and fat content stability), the pathophysiological mechanisms that lead to unintended weight gain maintenance, and the roles that excess weight and fat misdistribution play in contributing to chronic conditions such as diabetes, dyslipidaemia, heart disease, non-alcoholic fatty liver disease, and many others. As with other chronic illnesses, obesity originates from an interplay between an individual's genetic susceptibility to weight increase and environmental variables. Gene discovery in the area of weight control and obesity has revealed numerous important single-gene effects resulting in severe and early-onset obesity as well as many more minor genes with more varied effects on weight and fat distribution, including age-of-onset and severity. However, presently known main and minor genes explain only a tiny part of body weight variances in the population. Several environmental Contributors have also been recognised, but trying to counter these will probably require initiatives that fall far outside of the conversations taking place in the health care professional office between patient and provider since they involve making major societal changes regarding quality of food, work-related and leisure-time activities, and socio-economic factors including disparities in socio-economic status. Novel findings in disciplines of neuroendocrine and gastrointestinal regulation of hunger and energy expenditure have considerably progressed these studies in recent years. These discoveries have led to an expanding portfolio of drugs that, when combined with behavioural and lifestyle modifications, may help restore appetite control and enable moderate weight loss maintenance. They have also led to new processes that assist in explaining the improved results (both in terms of significant and sustained weight reduction as well as improvements or remission of co-morbid disorders) after bariatric surgeries such as laparoscopic sleeve gastrectomy and gastric bypass.

Chapter 1

Definition Of Overweight And Obesity

Overweight and obesity arise when excess fat storage (regionally, globally, or both) raises danger to health. It is the point at which health risk is elevated that is essential since, as detailed below, body weights and fat distributions that lead to the manifestation of co-morbid disorders occur at varied thresholds depending on the population.

Preferably, an obesity classification method would have the following features: it would be focused on a practical measurement commonly accessible to providers irrespective of their setting; it would correctly determine health risk (prognosis); it could be utilised to assign treatment strategies and goals. The most precise measures of body fat (the major component of body mass responsible for adverse outcomes) such as hydrostatic weighing, dual-energy x-ray absorptiometry (DEXA) scanning, computerised tomography

(C.T.), and magnetic resonance imaging (MRI) are impractical for use in everyday clinical occurrences.

Estimates of body fat, including body mass index (BMI, determined by dividing the body weight in kilograms by height in meters squared, or kg/m2) and waist circumference, do have constraints compared to these imaging techniques but still provide relevant information and are easily implemented in a variety of practice settings.

It is essential bringing out two significant limitations about thresholds used to identify overweight and obesity.

The first is that while we advocate the attribution of precise BMI cut-offs and rising risk, correlations between body weight or fat distribution and diseases that affect health really constitute a continuum. For example, increased risk for type 2 diabetes and early death begin much before a BMI of 30 kg/m2(the threshold to diagnose obesity in people of European extraction) is attained. It is in these early phases that preventive efforts to restrict additional weight gain and/or facilitate weight reduction will have their greatest health effects. The second is that traditional correlations between growing weight, weight, and co-morbidities are getting changed as new therapies for those disorders become available. For example, in the last few decades,

atherosclerotic cardiovascular (ASCVD) mortality has consistently dropped in the U.S. population, even while obesity rates have grown (see below) (see below). Although it is widely accepted that this decline in ASCVD deaths is due to better therapeutic interventions in the field (better coordination of "first responders" services such as ambulances and more prevalent use by the general populace of cardiopulmonary resuscitation and defibrillator units), through intensive care units, and in the office (statins, PCSK9 inhibitors, blood pressure medications, stents and other revascularisation procedures), these data have also been referenced to support of the claim that being overweight might actually protect against heart disease. In this context, updated epidemiological evidence on the health outcomes connected to being overweight or obese should include not

only statistics on morbidity and death but also health care use and expenses, including drugs and the number of treatment-related operations done.

Chapter 2
Consequences Of Obesity

You know that obesity is not healthy. You don't feel well, you don't look your best, and you may have begun to endure some of the health repercussions of being overweight. But what, precisely, are those consequences? Is being obese truly as harmful as many say? The top effects of obesity and being overweight, why it's crucial to your long-term health to begin a weight-reduction plan, health effects you'll escape by decreasing weight. Are you ready for some inspiration and motivation? Here, in no particular order, are the repercussions of obesity and being overweight over time.

1. Type 2 diabetes

When you are overweight, you're at a greater risk of being diagnosed with type 2 diabetes. Not everyone who is fat will have this condition, but a high number of individuals who have been diagnosed are, in fact, overweight.

Type 2 diabetes is commonly known as adult-onset diabetes. However, children may be diagnosed as well. And this sickness is nothing to laugh about! When you're diagnosed with type 2 diabetes, you'll experience an increase in thirst and numbness in your limbs. You may have repeated infections and sores that simply won't heal.

If left untreated, type 2 diabetes may be lethal. Amputations aren't uncommon, and blindness is a concern as well. In extreme circumstances, diabetic coma or death might result. Type 2 diabetes may be controlled with medicine and an improved lifestyle. But suffice to say, it's one of the most severe outcomes of obesity.

2. Bone and joint disease

When you're overweight, you're more likely to experience bone and joint damage. There are a number of explanations for this, but two are the most usually observed. First, obesity leads to reduced bone density. This creates fractures and bone disease.

Secondly, when you're fat, you're definitely not consuming the correct meals. A lack of sufficient nourishment will create difficulties with your bone health and may also lead to injury or bone disease.

Concerned about your joints? This one's straightforward - you're bearing greater weight on your joints. People who are obese are more prone to arthritis and other joint disorders as a consequence of their weight. Take action now and reduce weight so that you don't endure one of the most painful effects of obesity, bone and joint problems.

3. Heart disease

You may have previously known that one of the most prevalent outcomes of obesity is heart disease. Heart disease has quite a number of forms — here are a few:

- Enlarged ventricles which may induce heart failure
- Coronary artery disease
- High blood pressure
- High cholesterol
- Stroke
- Hypertension
- Angina

That's only to mention a few! When you're making your heart work harder, you're going to be at a larger risk for heart disease, plain and simple. As you're certainly aware, heart disease may be deadly.

4. Sleep apnea

Apnea is a condition in which a person stops breathing during sleep. Sound scary? It is. It's potentially risky for various reasons. First, of course, is that you're not breathing. You may wake up to find yourself struggling for air. The second is that sleep apnea substantially lowers the quality of your sleep.

People who suffer from sleep apnea find themselves lethargic and unable to focus throughout the day. Obviously, this might be rather risky while you're driving or if you're using machines at work. People who experience this consequence of obesity are also typically irritated, complain of regular headaches and report a reduction in the quality of their performance at work.

5. Cancer

Did you know that one of the effects of obesity is an increased risk of some forms of cancer? It's true, so all the antioxidants you've taken, and the sunscreen you've constantly applied may not assist you after all.

People who are overweight are more likely to be diagnosed with quite a few different forms of cancer. These include:

• Endometrial cancer

• Esophageal cancer

• Liver cancer

• Kidney cancer

• Pancreatic cancer

• Breast cancer (men, too) (men, too)

• Gallbladder cancer

Interestingly, obesity is associated with a cancer diagnosis but also with a prognosis. People who are obese are less likely to beat cancer than those who are a good weight. Furthermore,

people with a higher BMI are more likely to see cancer return once treated.Continue to apply sunblock and keep taking your antioxidants. But realise that keeping a healthy weight is also a good way to prevent cancer.

6. Metabolic syndrome

Metabolic syndrome has become one of those buzz terms you undoubtedly hear more regularly. In some respects, it's analogous to those who declare that their weight is a result of "thyroid problems." In some circumstances, that may be accurate. But in most, it's not.

While many individuals claim that metabolic syndrome is the reason they're fat, it's more probable that the contrary is true. Metabolic syndrome is precisely what the name implies: it's an incapacity of your metabolism to perform correctly. This may lead to high blood pressure, high triglycerides, diabetes or pre-diabetes and many other illnesses.

But make no mistake: you're not fat because you have metabolic syndrome. You have metabolic syndrome because you're fat. Losing weight and keeping a healthy lifestyle may lower the risks linked with metabolic syndrome and keep you healthy longer.

7. Psychological disorders

When you're fat, you're more likely to seek therapy for or be diagnosed with a psychiatric condition. We'll speak about depression in a bit. Right now, we're addressing various illnesses.

Studies have revealed that obesity has psychological implications, including:

• Dysthymia (chronic mild depression) (persistent mild depression)

• Agoraphobia (fear of leaving one's house or of crowds)

• Other specific phobias

• Anxiety

• Substance misuse includes drugs and alcohol

These illnesses are more likely to afflict women than males, but research isn't certain why.

Of course, there are certain very particular reasons why these mood disorders may be a result of the obesity you endure. For instance, bullying and ostracisation are regularly observed among fat persons. But while the study is still continuing, experts have positively associated obesity with an increased occurrence of psychiatric problems, independent of relationships.

8. Depression

When you're obese, you don't feel well. You feel physically weary, you don't feel good about yourself, and you may have extra pressures in your life that someone of normal weight does not. What's worse is that your prescription drugs for depression may actually induce weight gain, prolonging the cycle. There's no mistake about it that obesity has some major effects when it comes to your mental and emotional health. No of your age, it's easy to feel out of place, left out by others and just unhappy a lot of the time.

Depression is one of the most devastating effects of obesity.

Obesity is closely connected with an increase in suicide rates, especially in women and particularly those with a BMI higher than 40. If you are sad or have suicidal thoughts, please get assistance from a skilled professional.

9. Shorter life expectancy

We're not suggesting that you're going to die tomorrow as a result of fat. But it certainly does not improve your chances. Whether it's from cancer, heart disease, diabetes, liver or kidney disease or any other disorder, obesity has been proven to reduce your expected lifespan.

A study by the National Cancer Institute and the National Institutes for Health in the United States noticed adults from Australia, Sweden and the United States. The research revealed that those with a BMI of between 40 and 44.9 lost, on average, 6.5 years of life. Those with a BMI of 55 to 59.9 died a whole 13.7 years early than those with a healthy BMI.

Again, we're not saying you're certainly going to die younger than your healthy counterparts if you're obese. But this study sure does make you take a pause and think about whether trying to improve your lifestyle might be a good idea.

10. Infertility

If you're fat, you're more likely to be infertile than if you're healthy. And that's not all. If you're obese or overweight, you're less likely to carry a healthy baby to term than if you're healthy.

The reproductive implications of obesity are true for both men and women. Men, you're less likely to be able to establish a family if you're obese.

Women, you bear a broad spectrum of risks if you're overweight. You're more prone to experience gestational diabetes. Your conception and implantation rates plummet substantially. Your risk for miscarriage is considerably raised. And you're more likely to undergo miscarriage if you're obese.

These facts are true for both men and women, whether conception takes place spontaneously or with IVF. Even artificially inseminated couples endure loss and lack of success as a consequence of obesity.

11. Alzheimer's and dementia

Unfortunately, medicine has not yet led us to therapy for Alzheimer's. We don't know what causes it, and we don't know how to fix it. Alzheimer's and dementia are distressing to people who suffer from them and to the families who are left to care for them.

What we do know, however, is that obesity is directly connected to the risk for dementia. This is especially true for those persons who are obese between the ages of 40 and 60 years old. Science has not yet narrowed down the why of this, but then what is extremely evident.

Interestingly, scientists have gotten even more specific than BMI to determine risk factors for dementia. In summary, persons who are "thicker around the middle" are more likely to have dementia than those who merely have a higher BMI. They label this "centrally obese," and people who are classed as such are more likely to be diagnosed with Alzheimer's or dementia.

The struggle for early diagnosis and treatment of Alzheimer's is continuing. But we do know that you may minimise your chances of dementia by keeping a healthy weight.

12. Difficulty in movement

When you initially started to acquire weight, you undoubtedly realised that you weren't as "spry" as you formerly were. Sometimes it may have been difficult to rise up from a sitting posture on the floor. Then your boots were increasingly difficult to take on and fasten up. Now, you merely feel sluggish – maybe even ache – when you walk about.

You'll have good days, and you'll have awful days. But as a general rule, one of the effects of obesity is difficulties in moving. Your bones and joints will not be as healthy as they once were, and, of course, you're lugging quite a bit of additional weight around.

The good news is this: difficulties in mobility are nearly fully reversible. If you have problems with ordinary activities, don't worry.

You may make it better by just following a weight reduction strategy and exercising those muscles! Difficulty in mobility is hard to tolerate, but it's a long-term effect of obesity that may absolutely be overcome.

13. Digestive disorders

There are hundreds of digestive disorders that may be caused by fat. We'll only look at a handful here. First, we'd want to repeat that if you're fat, you're not eating appropriately. The nutrients you're putting into your body are substandard at best, and that might very well be the main cause of your digestive difficulties. Too many fats might make your bowel motions irregular. Too little fibre will go as well. If you're suffering digestive difficulties, consult a dietitian to fix what you can with a healthy diet.

That said, there are additional digestive diseases that are outcomes of obesity. To mention a few:

- Gastric ulcers
- Vomiting
- Bloating
- Heartburn
- Frequent diarrhoea
- Frequent constipation

If they seem unpleasant, they are! You may also endure extra flatulence and other humiliating concerns as a consequence of your fat. Protect your gut health and begin a weight reduction strategy to prevent this effect of obesity.

14. Inability to practice adequate hygiene

Ladies and gents, you know it's true. When you initially started to acquire weight, it got tougher and harder to wipe, wash, To reach down and trim your toenails. This is one of the most humiliating outcomes of obesity.

If you're reading this as a thin person, believe us when we tell you that even the most simple hygiene duties become considerably more challenging. Sure, it's simple to wash your face and brush your teeth. It's simple to put on makeup.

But it gets harder and difficult to reach back and brush your hair, much alone style it.

Even if you're using a back scrubber, getting around back there to wash your back gets challenging, wiping after the toilet gets harder. Shaving your legs? Forget it.

When you start getting heavier, the little hygiene acts you took for granted become much more difficult. Your appearance will alter, as will your distinctive aroma. Trust us when we tell you that this is a long-term effect of obesity that's not pleasant.

It can be harmful to you, as well. Bed sores are real, people, as are adult rashes and ingrown toenails. Do yourself a favour and start a weight reduction strategy to prevent this bad effect.

15. Discrimination

When you're obese, you're discriminated against. You could be passed over for the promotion. You may be compelled to purchase two aircraft tickets. You'll undoubtedly have to pay a "fat tax" at some time in your life - you know — increased pricing for plus-sized items. Discrimination is a very terrible but very real effect of fat. Can you do anything to alter it? Absolutely. You can get yourself on a weight-reduction plan and be one of the "skinny people.

But that's typically easier said than done, and what do you in the meantime? While you're busting your tail at the gym, at home, at your job, at school or all of the above, you're still having to deal with the thin crowd telling you you're not good enough.

For men and women, bullying is never appropriate. And you should never allow bullies to define your self-esteem and self-worth. Or body-shame you into believing you can't accomplish something you know you can. Your obesity is unhealthy, certainly. Work to improve it to develop a healthy lifestyle, but do not let it define you.

16. Higher medical expenditures

Alright. So, we touched on prejudice, but what about health costs? Is it fair, or is it right, for an insurance company to charge you a higher premium? For a doctor to charge you more, or for more tests, depending on your weight?

Yes. Absolutely.

As said, one of the effects of being fat is that you're more likely to die sooner. Hence the increased insurance prices. When you're obese, you may have underlying disorders that your doctor can't instantly identify as he might in a healthy person. That's literally the price you pay, and there's only one way to rectify it. Get on a healthy weight loss strategy.

As your BMI reduces, so will your medical bills. You'll be qualified for general insurance since you're no longer going to be high risk. Your physician can conduct some blood tests or otherwise check you and be able to narrow down the cause of your problem.

17. Respiratory disease

More and more, doctors and scientists are beginning to acknowledge that there's a relationship between obesity and respiratory disease. That said, this could be cyclical, and it's still yet unclear what that link is. See, if you have asthma, you'll be less inclined to go out and get the exercise you need. But is your obesity caused by asthma, or is your asthma caused by your obesity?

Obesity is definitely linked to sleep apnea, a respiratory condition. It's also directly connected to COPD. Obesity and asthma have been connected as well. Unfortunately, we don't yet have enough research to tell us which is the cause and which is the effect.

That However, if you're fat, you're more likely to be diagnosed with asthma, sleep apnea or COPD. Conversely, if you're a healthy weight, that danger lowers. So why not just bite the bullet and start a weight loss plan? You'll be less prone to experience respiratory illness, no matter the underlying association.

18. Lower quality of life

When you're obese, you can't go out and do activities as healthy individuals can. You're more likely to:

- Suffer depression
- Suffer anxiety
- Suffer persistent pain
- Be diagnosed with dementia
- Be discriminated against

And more

it only stands to reason that, as an obese person, you're going to have a lower standard of living. That's not to say you're without friends or fun. You just won't be able to enjoy your time in the exact way that a healthy person can.

Research performed by the North-western University Department of Medicine found that, as weight decreased, the psychological and physical lives of obese people improved. The reverse was also true – as weight increased, the social and physical well-being of such patients lessened.

If you've been overweight for some time, you may simply not remember how simple it was to go about your day and enjoy it. A weight-reduction plan can help you enhance the quality of your life as well as your longevity.

19. Social isolation

It's sad, but it's true. Obesity may lead to social isolation. Whether it's by choice or not, you may find yourself enjoying fewer trips, dating, social events and family reunions.

You can get yourself back on track. Again, don't ever allow a bully to define what you can and cannot do, but do take the comments of concerned family members to heart. They want you to live longer, feel better and be your best self.

Get out there, meet up with friends and get your weight reduction strategy on track. You don't have to feel alone anymore!

The disadvantages of obesity go well beyond merely not feeling or looking your best. There are several extremely significant long-term implications obesity will have on your health. Thankfully, most of these issues may be addressed pretty simply: just go out there and give it your best! Exercise, a healthy diet and a happy perspective will go a long way toward helping you prevent these repercussions!

Chapter 3
The Obesity Pandemic

The World Health Organization (WHO) 1997 recognised obesity as a serious public health concern and a worldwide epidemic. In general, a body mass index of 25 kg/m2 or above is considered overweight, and 30 kg/m2 or greater is considered obese. According to the estimations by WHO, more than 1.9 billion persons aged 18 years and older are overweight, and of them, over 650 million adults are obese.

Worldwide, the incidence of obesity has climbed rapidly throughout the previous four decades, and if this pattern continues, a majority of the global adult population will be either overweight or obese by 2030. Interaction of various elements, including genetic, metabolic, behavioural, and environmental impacts, has resulted in this predicament. The issue of obesity is a significant contribution to the worldwide burden of chronic illness and disability, with substantial social and psychological ramifications that impact practically all ages and socio-economic groups.

The main cause of various non-transmissible chronic medical illnesses and disability-adjusted life years worldwide, overweight and obesity, have reached pandemic proportions. Their widespread tendency is worsened by the prevalence of big socio-economic, ethnic, and environmental differences and by insufficient knowledge of the most beneficial and successful actions that may limit or reverse the path of the epidemic. To a large degree, these issues originate from the involvement of various individual, social, dietary, and environmental variables that impact the risk of obesity and overweight and shape the inequalities. This chapter gives a glance into a handful of these elements; there are many more, and some of them were likely not even discovered yet. If we evaluate these characteristics as a group, one of their most conspicuous qualities is their variety. Discrimination and racism, social capital, food environments, social networks, access to recreational facilities, and exposure to obesogens are the topics that historically belonged to separate disciplines yet are now consolidating into an intricate and dynamic interdisciplinary and cross-disciplinary network of acute medical, public, health, and economic relevance.

Adding to the present impact of the pandemic, emerging evidence points toward the potential of some of the major contributors to exert transgenerational effects, indicating that, in all likelihood, we have only witnessed the tip of the iceberg for what is increasingly being recognised as one of the greatest medical and public health challenges of our time.

Chapter 4
Why Obesity Has Risen

2.8 million people are predicted to die worldwide each year from obesity and overweight-related health issues, according to the World Health Organization (WHO) (WHO).

In a 2015 survey, CDC found 18.5 percent and 39.8 percent of American kids and adults, respectively, to be clinically obese (which indicates that their BMIs were 30 or greater) (which means that their BMIs were 30 or higher).

The incidence of obesity is much greater among older folks, with a recent Health Care Weekly article claiming the number of obese seniors in the U.S. has gone up by 36 percent in the previous one and half decades alone.

Obesity is the main risk factor for an array of chronic illnesses, such as heart disease, stroke, type 2 diabetes, arthritis, sleep apnea, hypertension, fatty liver disease, and at least three malignancies (endometrial, colon and breast cancer) (endometrial, colon and breast cancer).

There's little dispute obesity is an increasing problem for global public health. But why is it rising in practically every corner of the world? Here are science-backed explanations that can help explain the development of obesity globally.

1. Widespread Consumption of Processed and Junk Food

The issue with extensively processed meals is that they have little nutritional value. They are supposed to have a long shelf life, affordable and rather pleasant.

The difficulty is that food makers are tempting consumers to eat more low-quality junk food in an attempt to improve sales. The undesirable consequences include overeating, addiction, and the buildup of undesired fat.

Take MSG-infused, designed food items, for instance. They have little to no semblance to entire food. They are supposed to entice people to eat more and more, so packing calories that won't be utilised by the body and consequently end up being turned into extra weight.

In reality, most contemporary restaurants and retailers provide extensively manufactured meals that are enticing.

When paired with other environmental conditions, these food items induce overeating which leads to obesity.

2. Genetics Plays a Role

Some individuals are genetically prone to be overweight. In fact, multiple studies have shown that offspring of fat parents are more prone to acquire obesity later on. Don't get us wrong; obesity isn't fully dictated by heredity. Some environmental variables and changes in lifestyle could send weight growth signals to the genes, however.

In other words, heredity has some part in one's tendency to pack on weight but cannot be singularly accountable for obesity.

3. Insulin Resistance

Insulin is a crucial hormone that governs how fat is stored or utilised. Unfortunately, today's diet develops resistance to insulin. With higher quantities of insulin in the blood, more energy is turned into fat and stored rather than being utilised for metabolism.

While the subject is controversial, several studies have shown the link between obesity and high levels of insulin.

Thankfully, one can reduce insulin by cutting back on simple or refined sugars/carbs, as well as increasing the intake of dietary fibre.

4. Food Availability

Another reason why individuals are getting fat at a high rate is the availability of food, which has gone risen considerably globally in the previous several decades. More than two-thirds of the global population now eat at least three meals a day.

Another concern is that fast food is accessible everywhere, and it's growing cheaper by the day. On the contrary, complete foods and healthful meals are becoming unreasonably pricey.

For example, most individuals in disadvantaged neighbourhoods are unable to be able to purchase fresh vegetables and fruits. Meanwhile, big-box merchants and convenience stores provide them with packaged junk food, candy, drinks, and high-carb baked goods for a fraction of the price.

5. Added Sugar

Our contemporary diet is packed with Sugar, sweeteners, and other simple carbohydrates, including fructose, maltose, and glucose. The difficulty with ingesting large quantities of simple carbohydrates is that they impact our hormones and brain chemistry. In summary, it gets individuals addicted to Sugar, which adds to weight gain.

Even worse, a high fructose diet has been reported to induce elevated levels of blood insulin and insulin resistance. They also enhance appetite. And for this reason, extra Sugar in our diet promotes energy conversion to fat, which eventually leads to obesity.

Misinformation about health and diet can also lead to obesity. People are misled to accept trendy diets that yield no results. Poor knowledge may make weight reduction tougher and even lead to weight increase in certain situations.

How does Sugar tie in with the obesity epidemic?

Excessive unhealthy food and sugar-sweetened soft drink intake has been related to weight gain since it offers a substantial and needless source of calories with little or no nutritious value.

In 2010, WHO systematically commissioned a literature review to answer a series of questions relating to the effects of sugars on excess adiposity. These questions examined if lowering or increasing consumption of dietary sugars affects measures of body fatness in adults and children and whether the present data offer support for the advice to decrease intake of free sugars to less than 10% of total energy. Body fatness was chosen as an outcome in view of the degree to which co-morbidities of obesity contribute to the worldwide burden of non-communicable illness.

The conclusion of the meta-analysis reveals that the consumption of sugars is a factor of body weight in free-living persons eating ad libitum diets. The findings imply that the change in body fatness that happens with altering the consumption of sugars originates from a modification in energy balance rather than a physiological or metabolic consequence of monosaccharides or disaccharides.

Owing to the numerous reasons for obesity, it is predictable that the impact of lowering consumption is rather limited. However, when considering the quick weight gain that happens following increased consumption of sweets, it is plausible to infer that guidance pertaining to sugar intake is an important component of a plan to minimise the high risk of overweight and obesity in most nations.

Furthermore, the Scientific Advisory Committee on Nutrition (SACN) analysed randomised control studies, which demonstrated that intake of sugar-sweetened drinks, as compared with non-calorically sweetened beverages, resulted in weight gain and an increase in BMI in children and adolescents. Prospective cohort studies also largely corroborate the association between sugar-sweetened drinks and increasing adiposity.

6. Refined Carbohydrates

Carbs are an essential element of a balanced diet. Unprocessed carbohydrates include fibre, vitamins, and minerals. However, processing them eliminates nutrients and results in refined carbs, which people often refer to as empty carbs or empty calories.

Refined carbohydrates contain extremely few vitamins and minerals. The body absorbs refined carbohydrates rapidly, so they do not give sustained energy, and they may cause a person's blood sugar to jump.

In this post, we look at the distinctions between refined and complex carbohydrates. We also mention alternate meals that folks may pick.

What are they?

Bread produced from white flour is heavy in processed carbohydrates.

Carbs consist of:

• Sugars: Fruits, milk products, and ultra-processed meals, such as sodas and flavoured candy bars, contain sugars.

• Starches: Grains, legumes, and vegetables contain starches.

• Fibre: The digestive system cannot break down dietary fibre, which is found in fruits, vegetables, and other meals.

The body digests refined carbs fast, and they offer a source of energy. However, they may produce a fast spike in blood sugar and activate the pancreas to release insulin.

Big firms can also ultra-process food. The word ultra-processed denotes items that undergo manufacture on an industrial scale, such as soda and cookies.

Ultra-processed meals include elements that people do not use in normal cooking, such as additives.

They may have five times more added sugar than typical foods.

How do refined carbohydrates affect health?

The body consumes refined carbohydrates considerably more rapidly than it does unprocessed carbs.

As a consequence, refined carbohydrates generate a rapid burst of energy, but unprocessed carbs release energy more steadily throughout the day.

Once the brief burst of energy is done, a person may need to consume additional food to obtain more energy.

As a consequence, individuals might eat a significant quantity of calories, resulting in weight gain.

Having overweight or obese may raise the chance of health issues, such as:

- heart disease
- type 2 diabetes
- stroke
- hypertension
- asthma
- chronic backache
- osteoarthritis

Refined carbohydrates also do not have as much nutritious value as unprocessed carbs. They lack fibre, which is crucial for both digestive health and keeping blood sugar constant.

Chapter 5
The Calorie Anagram

Obesity in the U.K. remains at an all-time high. 64% of people throughout the U.K. are categorised as either overweight or obese, a rise of 11% in the previous 25 years. With more gyms, workout facilities, and access to personal trainers and nutritionists than ever, why are we still failing to lose weight as a nation?

Science tells us that reducing weight is quite uncomplicated. It's a straightforward computation of your calories in versus your calories out. If you consume more than you burn, you gain weight and vice versa. But is it that simple? And what additional forces are at play here?

BASICS OF CALORIES

Weight loss (and weight growth, for that matter) is largely a problem of calories; how many you eat and how much you expand. If the number of calories you consume and the number of calories you use each day are nearly the same, your weight won't change. It's only when you consume fewer calories than you use over a period of time that you will lose weight, and it's only when you eat more calories than you use that you will gain weight.

So, what amount of calories are we talking about? This is the fundamental calculation; one pound of body weight is equivalent to 3,500 calories. This implies that to lose one pound, you must generate a 3,500 calories-short by consuming fewer calories, burning more calories via physical exercise, or a combination of both. The exact reverse is true for weight gain, and it sounds a little like a lot, doesn't it? But it's not, actually. Gaining a pound is as simple as consuming an additional 250 calories a day (for instance, any of these; one chocolate bar, one bottle of soft drink, half a doughnut) for two weeks or missing a daily exercise without cutting down on eating.

A calorie is a calorie, whether it comes from protein, fat or carbohydrate (There are good calories and bad calories) (But there are good calories and bad calories).

Any calories ingested that your body doesn't burn for energy are deposited as body fat. No matter what sort of food box they came in.

There are a few more elements, in addition to calories, that impact your weight. They are your age, your gender, and your genetic blueprint. The one that matters most is your food consumption and physical exercise, therefore concentrate on these areas:

Calorie Count

Here's where the calories you consume come from. All are nutrients except alcohol, which offers just calories but no nutrition.

- 1 1 gram of protein offers four calories
- 1 1 gram of fat delivers nine calories
- 1 1 gram of carbohydrate delivers four calories
- 1 1 gram of alcohol delivers seven calories

Although you may be eager to lose weight as feasible, be cautious not to limit your daily calorie intake so much that you compromise your health. Women should not take in fewer than 1,200 calories a day when on a weight reduction diet, whereas males should consume no less than 1,800 calories a day (on a weight loss programme) (on a weight loss programme). It is challenging to receive all the vitamins and minerals you need each day when you lower your consumption below these quantities.

In fact, it's still challenging even at these calorie levels, so consider taking a daily multivitamin and mineral supplement. If you improve your physical activity level at the same time that you lower calories, you'll be able to take in a healthier and more fulfilling quantity of calories while still losing weight.

Little by little we're going further into the 'calories in' side of the equation, we notice how cultural norms may make it so simple to overeat, which can help us comprehend how all calories are not equal.

This often presents itself via tiny amounts of weight gain over the period of years until one day, we put on an old pair of pants, and it becomes tangible that we need to take action. The first thing to highlight is your upbringing. Your eating habits will most likely have been ingrained into your hardware from your parents. Were you ever rewarded with ice cream for excellent behaviour? Comforted with chocolate while you were sad? If this sounds similar, you could have gained an early adoption of emotional eating, which is widespread across the country and persists into maturity.

We also know that willpower and self-discipline don't always work, which is why your surroundings and the people you spend your time with will strongly affect your behaviour. Every day, we have a certain quantity of 'willpower energy', which is analogous to the battery on your phone. The longer you oppose something, the more this reserve of willpower declines. Traditional office-based professions these days are frequently loaded with cookies and chocolate, including entertaining customers with alcoholic lunches and late-night ordering while you're working on a project.

Making it through even just one day without all the excesses might be considered a triumph.

In addition to the foregoing, food of the current day has become highly accessible and pleasant. Hundreds of millions of pounds finance research that delves into the precise combinations that generate food products that are very gratifying and tap into our brain chemistry to crave more (ever stop after only three pringles...?). Coupled with the concept of 'mindless eating' where dining is no longer the daily ritual of breaking bread, engaging with people and savouring each mouthful.

On top of this combination of colourless food, our lives are getting busier. This may result in persistent tension and poor sleeping patterns, again leading to cravings and overeating. It has been demonstrated that persons who sleep fewer hours will have greater levels of hormones that influence sensations of fullness and hunger, fuelling a vicious cycle of increased desire and delayed sense of fullness. Coupled with heightened stress levels from working late hours or having a hectic family life, the main reaction of the body will be to resort to more coffee, more Sugar and more calories.

So, what can we do?

- **Regaining Control**

Planning ahead is usually a sensible option. How many of us come for lunch, hungry and empty-handed? Typically, that's where things go awry. This is the reason why Mark Zuckerberg wears the same thing every day. Psychologists believe that we all have a limited ability to make choices, and by eliminating a basic option such as what to dress, Mark is lowering any likelihood of 'decision fatigue later in the day on more complicated activities. From a dietary viewpoint, this may mean bulk cooking over weekends or employing a meal delivery service so that when Susan offers you cookies in the afternoon, you can simply say no.

Most new year's goals fail because there simply isn't any degree of responsibility involved. Having someone on board with you during your trip is one of the most crucial components of keeping motivation high and adhering to your commitment. This accountability might come from hiring a personal trainer or from something as easy as proclaiming your strategy to friends and family or to your social media following. Needless to say, this is something that you should be doing for yourself; however, having friends/family on board and/or a personal trainer who genuinely cares about your results will be a huge motivation.

Recognising the distinction between hunger and appetite is also fundamentally important for anyone who wishes to be successful in long-term weight management. Hunger can be described as a physiological need to eat to sustain life, whereas appetite usually refers to a hedonic desire for food. Eating to fuel performance and support optimal health should be our primary outlook on nutrition. This is where the advice of an expert is vital to guide you through the many phases of dieting, determine the ideal portion proportions, offer frequent feedback and help you build your nutrition I.Q. along the road.

The list below describes the essential basis of any effective strategy with an aim to encourage healthy weight reduction and support long-term weight control.

1. Exercising a minimum of 2-3x a week
2. Aiming to achieve 8000-10,000 steps a day
3. Getting 7-9 hours of sleep a night
4. Drinking enough water for your body
5. Eating a well-rounded diet that provides adequate macronutrient/micronutrients.

6. Supplementation, if required, to support increasing needs.

• **Putting it all together**

Weight loss can be a nerve-wracking idea for some and can provide many difficult obstacles along the way. Many of us have become victims of the downward spiral of health that comes with working long sedentary hours, hectic social lives and indulging too much on holidays. Our' calories in' side of the equation are constantly on a moving scale subject to the demands we place on our physiology, and as the years go by, our lack of proactivity will usually catch up to us.

Knowing you're 'why' will be one of your most valuable assets before commencing a weight loss journey. It could be that you're recently engaged and making plans for the big day. Or you're nearing a milestone birthday and want to be in the best shape of your life. Or it's a health-conscious act, and you're trying to protect yourself from cardiovascular disease as it runs in your family history. Whatever it may be, being equipped with this knowledge will accelerate you forward from the start line, pick you up if you fall down and spur you on through the finish line. Whether going alone or not, taking that initial step is the most critical step.

Chapter 6
The Hormonal Structure Of Obesity

Hormones are chemical messengers that govern activities in our bodies. They are factor in causing obesity. The hormones leptin and insulin, sex hormones and growth hormone regulate our hunger, metabolism (the rate at which our body consumes kilojoules for energy), and body fat distribution. People who are obese have levels of these hormones that encourage abnormal metabolism and the fat accumulation.

A system of glands, known as the endocrine system, secretes hormones into our bloodstream. The endocrine system works with the nervous system and the immune system to enables our body cope with different events and stresses. Excesses or deficits of hormones can lead to obesity, and, on the other hand, obesity can lead to changes in hormones.

- **Obesity and leptin**

The hormone leptin is created by fat cells and is released into our circulation. Leptin suppresses a person's appetite by working on certain areas of their brain to lessen their need to eat. It also appears to affect how the body controls its accumulation of body fat.

Because leptin is created by fat, leptin levels tend to be higher in people who are obese than in people of average weight.

However, despite having elevated levels of this appetite-reducing hormone, people who are obese aren't as sensitive to the impacts of leptin and, as a result, tend not to feel full during and after a meal. Ongoing research is looking at why leptin messages aren't getting through to the brain in people who are obese.

- **Obesity and insulin**

Insulin, a hormone produced by the pancreas, is critical for the control of carbohydrates and the metabolism of fat. Insulin stimulates glucose (Sugar) uptake from the blood in tissues such as muscles, the liver and fat. This is an important process to make sure that energy is available for everyday functioning and to maintain normal levels of circulating glucose.

In a person who is fat, insulin signals are occasionally lost, and tissues are no longer able to manage glucose levels.

This may lead to the development of type II diabetes and metabolic syndrome.

• **Obesity and sex hormones**

Body fat distribution has a crucial impact on the development of obesity-related illnesses such as heart disease, stroke and various kinds of arthritis. Fat around our belly is a larger risk factor for illness than fat accumulated on our bottom, hips and thighs. It appears that oestrogens and androgens contribute to determining body fat distribution. Oestrogens are sex hormones generated by the ovaries in pre-menopausal women. They are responsible for inducing ovulation every menstrual cycle.

Men and postmenopausal women do not generate much oestrogen in their testes (testicles) or ovaries. Instead, most of their oestrogen is created in their body fat, but at considerably lower quantities than what is produced in pre-menopausal ovaries. In younger men, androgens are produced at high levels in the testes. As a man gets older, these levels gradually decrease.

The changes with age in the sex hormone levels of both men and women are associated with changes in body fat distribution. While women of reproductive age prefer to store fat in their lower body ('pear-shaped'), older males and postmenopausal women tend to increase the storage of fat around their abdomen ('apple-shaped'). Postmenopausal women who are taking oestrogen supplements don't build fat around their midsection. Animal studies have also demonstrated that a lack of oestrogen leads to excessive weight gain.

• **Obesity and growth hormone**

The pituitary gland in our brain generates growth hormone, which regulates a person's height and helps develop bone and muscle. Growth hormone also impacts metabolism (the rate at which we burn kilojoules for energy) (the rate at which we burn kilojoules for energy). Researchers have shown that growth hormone levels in those who are fat are lower than in people of normal weight.

• Inflammatory factors and obesity

Obesity is also related to low-grade chronic inflammation inside the fat tissue. Excessive fat accumulation leads to stress responses inside fat cells, which in turn leads to the production of pro-inflammatory substances from the fat cells themselves and immune cells within the adipose (fat) tissue.

• Obesity hormones as a risk factor for illness

Obesity is related to an increased risk of a variety of disorders, including cardiovascular disease, stroke and numerous forms of cancer, and with reduced longevity (shorter life span) and worse quality of life. For example, the higher synthesis of oestrogens in the fat of older women who are obese is connected with an increase in breast cancer risk, demonstrating that the source of oestrogen production is crucial.

• Behaviour and obesity hormones

People who are obese have hormone levels that increase the storage of body fat. It appears that activities such as overeating and lack of regular exercise, over time, 'reset' the systems that govern hunger and body fat distribution to make the individual biologically more inclined to acquire weight. The body is continually attempting to maintain equilibrium, so it resists any short-term disturbances such as crash diets.

Various studies have revealed that a person's blood leptin level declines following a low-kilojoule diet. Lower leptin levels may increase a person's hunger and slow down their metabolism. This may help to explain why crash dieters frequently regain their lost weight. It is possible that leptin therapy may one day help dieters to maintain their weight loss in the long term, but more research is needed before this becomes a reality.

There is evidence to indicate that long-term lifestyle adjustments, such as a healthy diet and frequent exercise, may re-train the body to lose extra body fat and keep it off. Studies have also demonstrated that weight reduction as a consequence of a balanced diet and exercise or bariatric surgery leads to better insulin resistance, lower inflammation and favourable regulation of obesity hormones. Weight reduction is also related to a lower chance of getting heart disease, stroke, type II diabetes and several malignancies.

Chapter 7

Steps To Overcoming Obesity

1. Defeating Food Cravings:

For many of us working to lose or maintain weight, hunger isn't the largest issue we face. More often than not, it's desired. You can conquer food cravings! You don't have to be hungry to want certain meals. Unfortunately, naked carrot sticks or cauliflower don't evoke that "got to have it" sense for most of us.

So, how can we combat food cravings? You can accomplish that by understanding food desires.

Our desires nearly invariably lead us to food heavy in calories, fat, Sugar, and salt and poor in nutrients. Just denying a hunger might seem difficult. There are strategies to overcome those junk food cravings, maintain a balanced diet, and not feel so starved that you want to quit.

• Manage Your Stress

If you've ever found yourself "stress eating," there's a legitimate, physiological explanation. When you are under stress, your body boosts the production of the stress hormone. Cortisol boosts your blood sugar and inhibits insulin. This blocks the blood sugars from getting into the cells and makes the cells of the body feel "starved." The outcome is increased appetite and yearning for high-calorie meals. When you consume certain items, you feel better.

When you're feeling stressed out, sweet, fatty meals are literally a comfort.

To control your stress and halt this cycle in its track, consider exercising. The higher cortisol levels are there because your body is ready for fight or flight. So you're ready for a workout while you're anxious. Better still, many individuals find that a regular exercise regimen helps them avoid and reduce stress in the first place.

A less sweating option is meditation and deep breathing. Centring yourself and concentrating on your breathing may do wonders for relieving stress. You might also try spending a portion of your days on pastimes that you like. Life might feel incredibly hectic, but it's crucial to carve out some time for self-care. You may even discover that you're more productive the remainder of the day after you've taken your mind off your difficulties by indulging in an activity you like simply for the enjoyment of it.

Another wonderful alternative is to consult a therapist for assistance in managing stress. Just expressing your troubles with a neutral person may help make them more bearable, and a competent counsellor can also provide you with some specific advice and tactics to help you decrease stress.

• Get Your Sleep

Poor sleep doesn't simply leave you irritable and weary. It leaves you famished. Have you ever felt hungrier than usual after a night of less-than-great sleep? There's a reason. Lack of sleep raises the hunger hormone ghrelin. And reduces the hunger-diminishing hormone leptin. This combo leaves your body in need of some rapid energy. Combine that with the impaired decision-making skills that lack of sleep also produces, and you've got a formula for some major junk food eating.

To lessen junk food cravings, improve your sleep patterns.

That includes avoiding coffee, alcohol, or heavy meals before night. And just like with children, adults benefit from a nightly schedule as well. Avoid devices and ease into rest with low lighting and stillness. Once you have a routine established, your body will recognise the cues that it's bedtime and start getting ready for sleep.

• Stay On Top of Your Meal Times and Eat Enough

If you spend too long without eating, your blood sugar level will plummet. That sends a message to your body that you need energy, and you need it immediately. The fastest energy is Sugar, so that's usually what you'll find yourself needing if you allow your blood sugars to sink too low. You consume junk food, your blood sugar climbs, causing more insulin to be produced, and before you know it, you're on the blood sugar roller coaster.

The easiest method to guarantee that you're eating healthy and frequently is to perform meal prep and planning once a week.

That way, you aren't left attempting to figure out what's for supper when you're tired and hungry. Choose lean proteins, healthy fats, fibre, and complex carbohydrates.

Just as crucial as what you eat is avoiding missing meals. You should eat every 2.5 to 3 hours. That doesn't imply a complete meal, but a healthy snack to maintain your blood sugars consistent and level can do wonders for minimising your cravings.

• Avoid the "All or Nothing" Mentality

Avoid placing yourself on a tight "diet" that focuses on what you can't have. Instead, strive for a healthier lifestyle with better food choices that you can live with over a longer length of time, and don't deprive yourself of a treat if you absolutely want one.

An all-or-nothing mentality might set you up for cravings.

No one likes to fear they'll never eat a favourite meal again. Go ahead and pamper yourself, but do it thoughtfully. Have a single modest scoop of ice cream, don't simply grab a carton and a spoon. You'll appreciate it more, and it won't come with the waves of remorse that follow accidentally striking the bottom of the container.

• Drink water

Your body is incredibly clever about a lot of things, yet it commonly confuses thirst for hunger. If you're drinking water throughout the day, you're less likely to let your body make that mistake.

Besides the uncertainty about what your body truly requires, dehydration produces weariness, which promotes cravings.

Just like with lack of sleep, dehydration and weariness make your body craving for a rapid boost of energy. If you have a desire, drink a glass of water and wait 10 minutes. You may discover that hunger vanishes.

• Eat Probiotics

Your desires aren't all in your brain! Some of them originate from your gut. That's accurate; the microbial balance in your stomach may boost desires, particularly for sweets. The bacteria that you feed is the bacteria that will grow in your stomach. If you routinely consume processed, sugary meals, the bacteria that feed on such foods can colonise the stomach and may lead to the desire for those high-sugar items.

Keeping things balanced and stocking your stomach with the "good bacteria" is a key impact in minimising cravings.

You may acquire a range of healthful types of probiotics by consuming fermented foods like yoghurt, kefir, tempeh, kimchi, kombucha, and even pickles.

If you want to go for a probiotic supplement, examine the strain kinds and quantities. Lactobacillus Acidophilus and Bifid bacterium have been related to a decrease in desires. Also, check for a count of over 10 billion viable cells/colony-forming units. Some formulations I prescribe to my patients are I flora, Ultimate Flora, and Flor advantage.

• Medications

If you are still battling junk food cravings, speak to your bariatrician or doctor about drugs that may help you break the habit and get into a better pattern.

Sometimes just that small support is all you need to make life adjustments to enhance your health!

2. Exercise regularly

Obesity results from energy imbalance: too many calories in, too few calories burned. A lot of variables determine how many calories (or how much "energy") individuals burn each day, among them age, body size, and DNA.

But the most changeable factor-and, the most readily modified, is the number of movements individuals receive each day.

Keeping active may help individuals remain at a healthy weight or lose weight. It may also cut the risk of heart disease, diabetes, stroke, high blood pressure, osteoporosis, and some malignancies, as well as relieve stress and increase mood. Inactive (sedentary) lives do quite thc opposite. Despite all the health advantages of physical movement, people worldwide are doing less of it-at work, at home, and as they travel from place to place. Globally, around one in three persons receives little, if any, physical exercise. Physical activity levels are dropping not just in wealthier nations, such as the U.S., but also in low- and middle-income countries, such as China. And it's obvious that this loss in physical activity is a fundamental factor in the worldwide obesity pandemic, and in turn, in growing rates of chronic illness everywhere.

The World Health Organization, the U.S. Dept. of Health and Human Services, and other experts say that for excellent health, individuals should acquire the equivalent of two and a half hours of moderate-to-vigorous physical exercise each week. (2–4) Children should receive much more, at least one hour a day. There's been some discussion among academics, though, regarding precisely how much movement individuals need each day to maintain a healthy weight or to aid with weight reduction, and the most current studies show that a total of two and a half hours a week is just not enough.

3. Consider dieting

It's no secret that the quantity of calories individuals consume and drink has a direct influence on their weight: Consume the same number of calories that the body burns over time, and their weight remains steady. Consume more than the body burns, and weight goes up. Less, weight goes down. But what about the type of calories: Does it matter whether they come from specific nutrients-fat, protein, or carbohydrate? Specific foods-whole grains or potato chips? Specific diets-the Mediterranean diet? And what about when or where people consume their calories: Does eating breakfast make it easier to control weight? Does eating at fast-food restaurants make it harder?

There's substantial evidence on foods and eating patterns that protect against heart disease, stroke, diabetes, and other chronic illnesses. The good news is that many of the foods that help prevent illness also tend to assist with weight control foods like whole grains, vegetables, fruits, and nuts. And several of the items that enhance illness risk-chief among them, refined grains and sugary drinks-are also contributors to weight gain. Conventional wisdom states that because a calorie is a calorie, regardless of its source, the best advice for weight management is simply to eat less and exercise more. Yet recent evidence shows that certain foods and eating behaviours may make it easier to keep calories in control, while others may make individuals more inclined to overeat.

4. Consider considering a weight loss operation. Weight loss surgery, also called bariatric or metabolic surgery, is sometimes used as a treatment for individuals who are very obese and can lead to significant weight loss and help improve many obesity-related conditions, such as type 2 diabetes or high blood pressure.

But it's a huge operation and, in most cases, should only be considered after trying to lose weight through a healthy lifestyle and regular exercise. There are various forms of weight loss surgery.

The most common types are:

- Gastric band — a band is put around your stomach, so you do not need to eat as much to feel full.
- Gastric bypass – the top part of your stomach is joined to the small intestine, so you feel fuller sooner and do not soak up as many calories from food.
- Sleeve gastrectomy – some of your stomach is removed, so you cannot eat as much as you could before, and you'll feel full sooner.

All these surgeries may lead to considerable weight reduction within a few years, but each has pros and downsides.

If you're contemplating weight reduction surgery, talk to a surgeon about the numerous kinds available to help determine which is best for you.

Risks of weight loss surgery

Weight loss surgery poses a minor risk of problems.

These include:

- Being left with superfluous folds of skin - you may require subsequent surgery to remove them, and it is not typically given free of charge. Not obtaining enough vitamins and minerals from your food — you'll probably need to take supplements for the rest of your life following surgery.
- Gallstones (small, hard stones that form in the gallbladder) (small, hard stones that form in the gallbladder)
- a blood clot in the leg (deep vein thrombosis) or lungs (pulmonary embolism) (pulmonary embolism)
- the gastric band falling out of position, food spilling from the junction between the stomach and small intestine, or the gut being plugged or constricted

Before having surgery, talk to your surgeon about the possibilities.

Conclusion

Obesity is among the most frequent illnesses in the contemporary world. As such, it is crucial to find out what variables both contribute to and lessen the risk of being overweight or obese. This research has done so by utilizing real obesity data in place of the self-reported data that has been utilized in most prior obesity studies done in Canada. Using Moran's I and K-analyses, it was shown that there does not seem to be an association between parks and obesity rates nearby. However, the findings of the Point Density study contradict that.

More research must be undertaken at a better resolution to uncover how the built environment influences obesity rates and to identify precisely how walkability may affect Obesity rates. Whether there is a connection that individuals of normal weight distribution live near parks and relocate to where there are parks and open access, or whether people who are overweight and obese are utilizing these institutions to lose weight.

Further study undertaken after acquiring all the required data may aid to lessen the number of restrictions found throughout this endeavour. Comparison research evaluating the variations between the findings obtained from different places might be useful in defining the most relevant environmental risk factors involved in the prevalence of Obesity.

www.ingramcontent.com/pod-product-compliance
Lightning Source LLC
LaVergne TN
LVHW052055160826
845678LV00015B/3244